Stem Cells

for

Osteoarthritis

Treatment

Discover the "inside" secrets

By,

Nathan Wei, MD, FACP, FACR

www.arthritistreatmentcenter.com

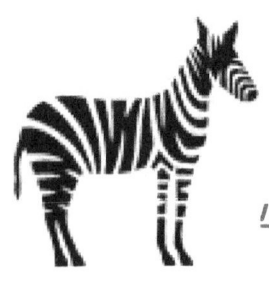

／.arthritistreatmentcenter.com

electronic or mechanical including recording, duplicating, or by informational storage or retrieval system without the written permission from the author and publisher.

This book should not be a substitute for a thorough examination by your physician. The products that are mentioned in this book are recommended. Prior to using any of them, we recommend you seek advice from a qualified specialist. Neither the publisher nor the author may be held liable for any injury, loss, or damage sustained by anyone who relies on the information contained in the book.

Table of Contents

www.arthritistreatmentcenter.com

Chapter 1

Osteoarthritis – An expensive condition…

Osteoarthritis is on the increase, with more than 27 million Americans currently affected -- a number that is expected to swell to 67 million by 2030.

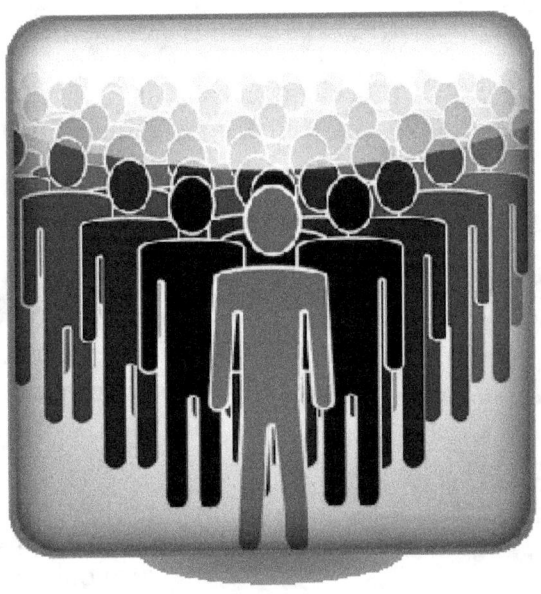

www.arthritistreatmentcenter.com

People with osteoarthritis suffer from loss of cartilage in weight-bearing areas of the skeleton including the knees, hips, hands, feet and spine.

Medical care for osteoarthritis patients in the United States costs **$185.5 billion a year**, according to a new study, published in the December 2009 issue of Arthritis & Rheumatism.

Of that amount, insurers pay $149.4 billion while patients pay $36.1 billion in out-of-pocket costs. Annual insurer costs are $4,833 per female patient and $4,036 per male patient. Women also have higher out-of-pocket expenses than men -- $1,379 versus $694. The total cost for female patients is $118 billion, compared with $67.5 billion for male patients.

"…Our study clearly reflects the significant impact of OA on U.S. healthcare spending," commented study author John Rizzo, of Stony Brook University in New York.

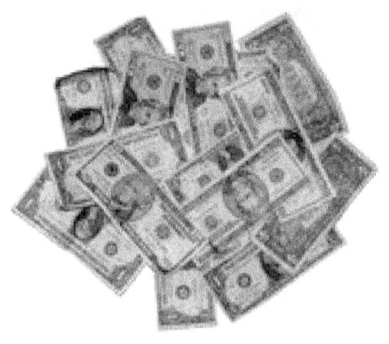

Annual expected aggregate healthcare expenditures relating to osteoarthritis increased dramatically each year:

One shortcoming of the study calculations is that the study included only direct medical costs, such as physician, hospital, and outpatient services, but did not consider other expenditures such as physical and occupational therapy. Undoubtedly, the price tag would be much higher, otherwise.

Rizzo and his colleagues analyzed 1996-2005 data from the Medical Expenditure Panel Survey. The data sample included 84,647 women and 70,590 men aged 18 and older who had health insurance. The healthcare costs included physician, hospital and outpatient services, as well as drugs, diagnostic tests and related medical services.

The study authors said increased awareness and better screening to identify patients with osteoarthritis may help delay disease progression and resulting disability, thus reducing medical costs.

"Our results suggest that patients with OA may benefit from greater efforts to promote exercise, proper medication use and appropriate surgical treatments for the disease," Rizzo concluded.

"Understanding the economic costs of osteoarthritis is important for payers, providers, patients, and other stakeholders," underscored the researchers.

As the Baby Boomer demographic ages, these figures will undoubtedly grow larger.

Chapter 2

Osteoarthritis: The basic biology

The "gristle" that caps the ends of long bones is called cartilage. It is this gristle that allows the surfaces of long bones to interact or articulate. Under normal circumstances, the articular surfaces of a normal joint are smooth and glistening.

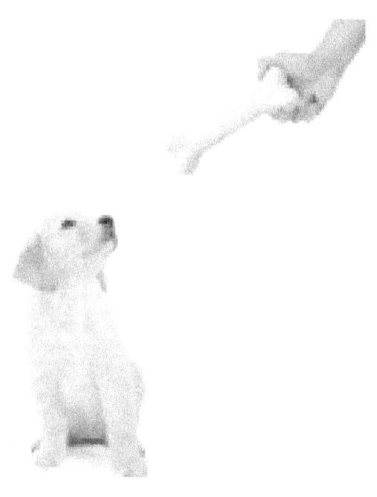

In osteoarthritis, the cartilage is thin, eroded, and discolored. Bone spurs, called osteophytes grow.

Type 2 collagen fibers, which are made up of a triple helix of amino acid chains with a unique composition, contribute to the strength and structure of articular cartilage (Kang AH. Connective tissue: collagen and elastin, in Kelley WN, Harris ED Jr., Ruddy S, Sledge CB (eds:. Textbook of Rheumatology. Philadelphia, WB Saunders Company 1981, pp 221-238).

Collagen fibers are anchored in the bone beneath the cartilage. Packed between the collagen fibers are groups called proteoglycans. These proteoglycans are loaded with water and tend to expand between the collagen fibers (Myers ER, Mow VC. Biomechanics of cartilage and its response to biomechanical stimuli, in Hall BK (ed): Cartilage, Volume 1 Structure, Function and Biochemistry. New York, Academic Press, 1983, pp 313-341.

A proteoglycan group or aggregate consists of a long chain of hyaluronic acid, along which individual proteoglycan molecules are attached (Rosenberg L: Structure of cartilage proteoglycans, in Burleigh PMC, Poole AR (eds): Dynamics of Connective Tissue Macromolecules. North-Holland Publishing Company, Amsterdam, 1984, pp 105-128).

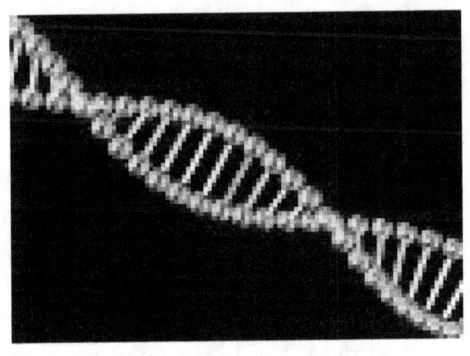

This is what a chain of hyaluronic acid looks like.

A proteoglycan molecule contains two types of glycosaminoglycans: chondroitin sulfate and keratin sulfate. A large number of these proteoglycan molecules are attached to a single hyaluronate strand forming a large aggregate. This large complex binds water. The electrical charges within this complex prevent water from flowing out when subjected to compression. Therefore, cartilage remains elastic (Witter JM, Roughley PJ, Webber C, et al. Arthritis Rheum 1987; 30: 519-529).

When cartilage is compressed during normal activity, the electrical charges within the proteoglycan complex resist.

Articular cartilage has no blood vessels or nerves. All components of articular cartilage are manufactured by the chondrocyte, the only cell present within normal cartilage.

The chondrocyte is active metabolically and makes a variety of enzymes concerned with maintaining the integrity of cartilage.

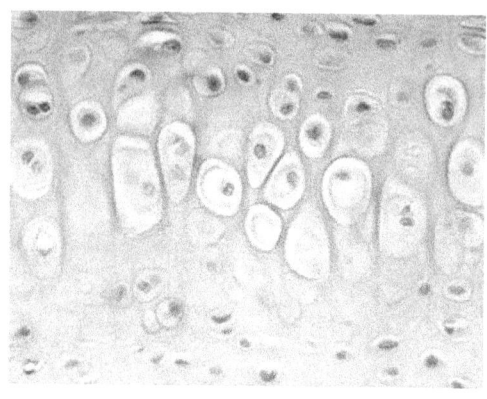

Chondrocytes

Cartilage metabolism becomes disrupted in osteoarthritis. The earliest change in cartilage when it develops osteoarthritis is an increase in water content. This occurs because of a defect in the collagen network that allows proteoglycans to absorb more water. As osteoarthritis progresses, proteoglycans become abnormal and decrease in number. A decrease in keratin sulfate with an increase in chondroitin sulfate occurs.

Cartilage begins to soften and the surface frays and splits. This process is termed fibrillation.

Also, chondrocytes begin to produce and release destructive enzymes such as hyaluronidase, cathepsin D, proteinases, lysosomal enzymes, and collagenase.

Chondrocytes do make an attempt to repair damage by increasing their metabolic rate and synthesizing more collagen and proteoglycan, but soon destruction outweighs repair.

www.arthritistreatmentcenter.com

At the same time, the cells in the synovium begin to make destructive enzymes that contribute to the breakdown of cartilage.

Chapter 3

How does osteoarthritis develop and what can you do to treat it?

Cartilage is a tough, flexible connective tissue that is found throughout the body. This rubbery tissue which covers the ends of long bones functions mainly as a cushion for joints. Because it is covered by a thin layer of lubricating material called "synovial fluid," it also acts to allow gliding of joints.

Cartilage does not have a blood or nerve supply... as a result, unlike damaged skin or muscles or other organ systems that can heal, damaged cartilage early on is not associated with pain and does not heal quickly.

There are three types of cartilage:

- Elastic cartilage is a pliable form of cartilage found in structures such as the outside of the ears, nose, and epiglottis.
- Fibrocartilage is a tough type of cartilage and is very shock resistant. It is found in the discs that form part of the spinal column and also is the type of cartilage that makes up the meniscus (ring of cushion material) located in the knees, hips, and shoulders.

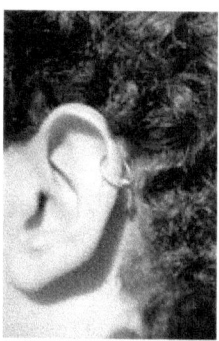

Elastic cartilage

www.arthritistreatmentcenter.com

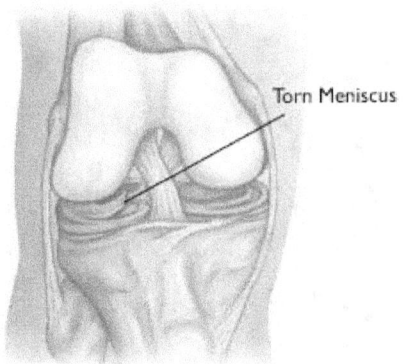

Torn Meniscus

- Hyaline cartilage is a softer type of cartilage that is found most commonly in joints.

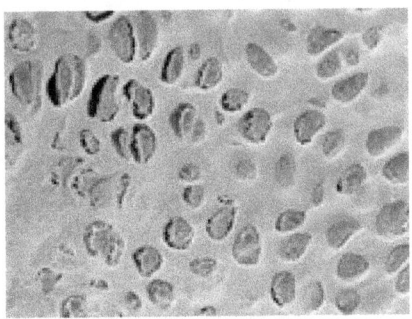

Hyaline cartilage

Cartilage damage is not painful early on, as mentioned earlier, since no nerve fibers are present. However, as the problem progresses and develops into arthritis, there are symptoms which do occur.

A 12-year study in middle-aged adults suggests that knee pain is frequently the first sign of knee osteoarthritis.

www.arthritistreatmentcenter.com

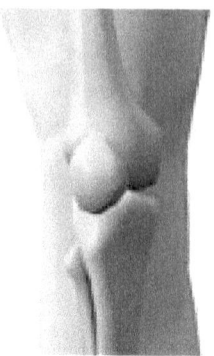

"Knee pain is common and may well be an early feature of knee osteoarthritis," lead author Dr. C. A. Thorstensson, from the Research and Development Center, Oskarstrom, Sweden, and colleagues write, "but studies to confirm the relationship are sparse."

The study featured 143 adults with knee pain lasting for longer than 3 months. These individuals were members of the population-based Spenshult cohort.

Weight-bearing x-rays of the knees had been taken at baseline and again at 12 years.

"A majority of middle-aged patients with chronic idiopathic knee pain in this study developed knee osteoarthritis over 12 years," the authors state. On this basis, they conclude, "Knee pain is often the first sign of knee osteoarthritis." (*Ann Rheum Dis* 2009;68:1890-1893).

Symptoms of articular cartilage damage include:

- decreased range of movement in the affected joint
- joint pain
- stiffness with inactivity
- swelling

If the damage is particularly severe, a piece of cartilage can break off and become loose. In this case, the loose piece of cartilage may affect the movement of the joint. This can cause a feeling of 'locking' or 'catching'. Sometimes, the joint may also give way.

www.arthritistreatmentcenter.com

Articular cartilage damage can occur as a result of trauma- a direct blow to the cartilage. This is why cartilage damage is often a problem for people who play contact sports.

Cartilage can also become damaged gradually, over time. There is an increased risk of developing this type of cartilage damage for heavy individuals, or for people with an anatomic abnormality which causes a structural problem with the joint.

Interestingly enough, immobility can also damage the cartilage.

The major problem when damage occurs to cartilage is that articular cartilage has a very limited capacity for self repair. A small amount of damage does not repair itself and often gets worse over time.

The diagnosis of cartilage damage can be suspected by a careful history and physical examination. Confirmation can be obtained by diagnostic studies such as:

- Magnetic resonance imaging (MRI): MRI scans use strong magnetic fields to produce detailed images of the inside of the body. It can often detect cartilage damage.
- Diagnostic ultrasound: This relatively new method of musculoskeletal diagnosis uses sound waves to image cartilage and inflammation.
- Arthroscopy: This is a form of surgery where an arthroscope, a small telescope, is used to look inside the joint.
- X-ray: While this is the traditional method of imaging, the drawback is that osteoarthritis has to be relatively severe before it shows up on x-ray.

There are a number of treatments that can help to relieve the symptoms of damaged articular cartilage.

www.arthritistreatmentcenter.com

Nonsurgical approaches include:

- Non-steroidal anti-inflammatory drugs (NSAIDS) help with pain and inflammation. They do have potential side effects that require close monitoring.
- Physical therapy. Various types of treatments such as electrical stimulation, diathermy, and ultrasound may reduce pain. Exercises which strengthen the muscles supporting the joint may help to reduce the pressure on the joint, and reduce pain.
- Assistive devices. Canes, walkers, and braces are sometimes useful.
- Lifestyle changes. Weight reduction, regular exercise, and so on can be useful.
- Corticosteroid injections can reduce pain and swelling temporarily but should not be given in the same joint more than 3 times per year.
- Viscosupplements are special lubricants that may dramatically improve pain and mobility when injected into a joint. It is strongly recommended that steroid and viscosupplement injections be given using ultrasound guidance to ensure proper placement of injections.

When non-surgical approaches aren't enough, then surgical treatments may be required.

Arthroscopic lavage and debridement employs an arthroscope to wash the joint out. The technique cannot repair the damaged cartilage, but it can help to reduce the pain and increase mobility.

Microfracture surgery: This is a procedure that involves drilling tiny holes (micro fractures) into the bone underneath the damaged cartilage. This exposes the blood vessels inside the bone. Blood cells then begin to stimulate the production of new cartilage. The disadvantage is that the newly formed cartilage is fibrocartilage rather than hyaline cartilage. Fibrocartilage is not as strong as hyaline cartilage. Therefore, it can wear away more quickly than hyaline cartilage.

Mosaicplasty: This is a technique that involves removing healthy cartilage from the non-weightbearing areas of a joint and using it to replace damaged cartilage.

Autologous chondrocyte implantation (ACI): This is a technique where a small sample of cartilage cells is taken from the non-weight bearing part of the knee. The cells are sent to a laboratory where they are stimulated to divide and produce new cells. After a few weeks, the number of cartilage cells will have increased by about 50-100 times from their original number. The new cartilage cells will then be placed under a flap of material that is sewn over the damaged part of the joint.

For patients where cartilage has worn away completely, total joint replacement is probably the procedure of choice. While it is successful for most people, there are potential complications such as infection, blood clots, and prosthesis failure which can occur.

There are a number of research projects that are currently investigating additional efficient and effective ways of repairing cartilage.

- Hybrid cartilage is an investigational procedure where human cartilage cells are combined with synthetic fibers to form a patch.
- Stem cells: Another area of research is looking at ways of using special cells, known as stem cells, to generate new cartilage. This latter procedure is promising. Unfortunately, only a few centers worldwide have the knowledge and expertise to perform this procedure properly.

www.arthritistreatmentcenter.com

Chapter 4

Current concepts in osteoarthritis research: So why do my knees hurt and can you make them better?

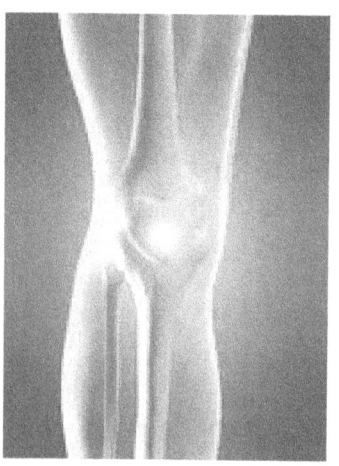

Osteoarthritis (OA) is one of the most common conditions leading to disability and impaired quality of life in the Western world.

Ironically, while more effective disease-modifying therapies have been developed for rheumatoid arthritis, particularly within the last 10-15 years, rheumatologists still treat osteoarthritis with symptomatic and supportive therapies.

As a result, the inexorable progression of this disease results in the performance of more than half a million joint replacements annually in the United States. While joint replacement surgery has made gigantic strides, it is still a major surgical procedure.

www.arthritistreatmentcenter.com

Risk factors for the development of OA include: genetic factors, obesity, joint injury, surgery, and the presence of associated metabolic disease.

It is clear from the research that OA is a disease that involves not only the cartilage- the gristle that caps the end of long bones and cushions the joint, but also the synovium- the tissue lining the joint- as well as the bone that underlies cartilage.

While genetic factors play a significant role in the incidence of osteoarthritis, the damage that occurs is a result of a complex interaction of inflammatory messengers. Among these are cytokines, prostaglandins, nitric oxide, growth factors, and proteases.

These substances, which are produced by chondrocytes (cartilage cells) that are subjected to abnormal forces lead to a situation where there is premature aging and destruction of cartilage substance.

The production of these inflammatory proteins also contributes to inflammation of the synovium and excessive amounts of bone growth.

Present therapies, as issued by guidelines proposed by the Osteoarthritis Research Society International (OARSI), are clearly aimed at symptom relief. These treatments include: analgesics, non-steroidal anti-inflammatory drugs (NSAIDS), topical agents ("rubs"), and joint injections with either glucocorticoids ("cortisone"), or hylauronic acid lubricants.

Current research has been aimed at finding the triggers that cause inflammation to start and also to identify specific markers that might identify those patients who are at greatest risk for rapid progression of disease. These markers would also be useful in measuring improvement once newer drugs that can slow down disease progression in OA can be discovered.

www.arthritistreatmentcenter.com

However, all of these investigations are futile unless and until specific disease-modifying osteoarthritis drugs (DMOADS) – drugs that slow down the rate of cartilage loss- can be developed.

Drugs aimed at inhibiting cytokine and protease function show some promise but it is still too early to tell whether they will have the desired effect. Examples of these drugs include: matrix metalloproteinase inhibitors, drugs that block interleukin 1, bisphosphonates, calcitonin, as well as nutritional supplements such as glucosamine and chondroitin.

And it may not be enough to find drugs that simply slow disease progression.

The "holy grail" is still the treatment(s) that will rebuild cartilage. The type of therapy that shows the greatest promise to date is the use of autologous stem cells. These are stem cells harvested from the patient and reintroduced into the affected joint along with a specific matrix to which the stem cells can adhere and grow.

Chapter 5

Why settle for "Golden Year Knees" when "Glory Year Knees" are possible?

How can some people defy aging joints while their knees keep getting older every day? What would you do to have knees that were 20 years younger? If you had knees that were 20 years younger, what would you do first?

Maybe go for a long bike ride... run a 10 K race... or simply take your granddaughter to the zoo without dreading the thought of struggling up and down steps or curvy hilly pathways...

Is it possible to control the aging process of osteoarthritis and reverse its negative effects on weight-bearing joints such as the knees?

The answer may surprise you.

Osteoarthritis is the most common form of arthritis - it's estimated that perhaps 30 million people in the United States suffer from the condition.

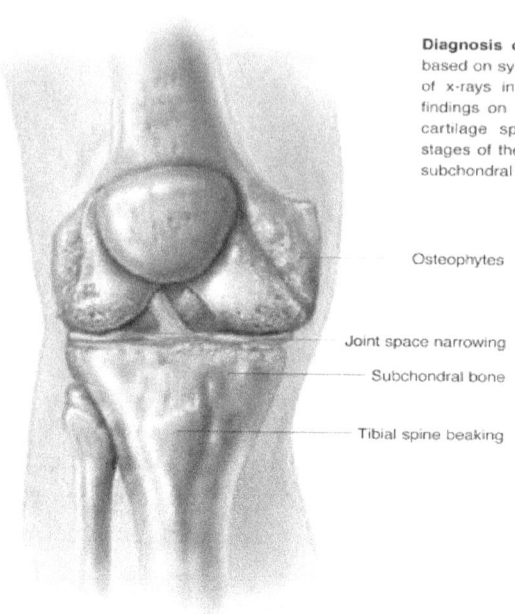

Diagnosis of osteoarthritis of the knee is based on symptoms and signs, and on results of x-rays in asymptomatic patients. Positive findings on radiographs include narrowing of cartilage space (mostly unilateral in early stages of the disease), marginal osteophytes, subchondral sclerosis, and tibial spine beaking.

Osteophytes

Joint space narrowing

Subchondral bone

Tibial spine beaking

Osteoarthritis is a disease caused by "wear and tear". The cartilage – the cushion – at the end of long bones erodes away prematurely and becomes thinner and rougher leading to narrowing of the joint space. Subchondral bone (the bone underneath the cartilage) compensates by getting thicker and growing outwards beyond the joint. This process causes the formation of bony spurs, called "osteophytes." Other bony sites begin to grow and start to get "pointy." This is sometimes referred to as "beaking."

Symptoms of osteoarthritis include stiff, swollen, painful joints. As the condition progresses, the joints become deformed and knobby.

In a study reported in the Annals of the Rheumatic Diseases in 2006, osteoarthritis may be a sign of faster "biological aging." The authors based their findings on a study of almost 1100 people, aged between 30 and 79. The authors suggested that both the aging process and

www.arthritistreatmentcenter.com

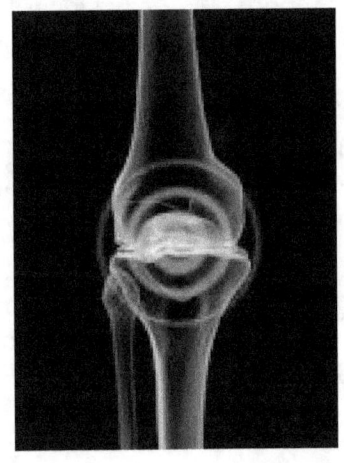

osteoarthritis share biological factors in common, including oxidative stress and low level chronic inflammation.

The field of regenerative medicine has long believed that adult stem cells have the potential to significantly protect and possibly regrow cartilage in conditions such as knee osteoarthritis.

Many studies have been conducted both in large animals as well as humans.

One such project was conducted at the Murdoch School of Veterinary and Biomedical Sciences (Australia).

Murdoch's cartilage trials evaluated the effectiveness and safety of allogeneic adult stem cells to treat osteoarthritis of the knee in 48 arthritic sheep joints.

The results showed that osteoarthritic sheep knee joints receiving stem cells had significantly greater thickness of joint cartilage, reduced cartilage breakdown, and greater biomechanical strength three months later than did control joints.

Professor Rick Read, lead investigator stated, "We are delighted with the significant cartilage protective effects of ...allogeneic (donor unrelated) cells in our large animal model of knee osteoarthritis, without any adverse events of the cells at all..."

A Cardiff University (U.K.) study has lent credence to the idea that stem cell therapy should be studied in humans.

www.arthritistreatmentcenter.com

Lead researcher Professor Charlie Archer reports, "We have identified a cell which, when grown in the lab, can produce enough of a person's own cartilage that it could be effectively transplanted."

He goes on to say, "This research could have real benefits for arthritis sufferers and especially younger active patients with cartilage lesions that can progress to whole scale osteoarthritis."

Scientists at the Scripps Institute in La Jolla, California have shown how the loss of the protein HMGB2, found in the surface layer of joint cartilage, leads to the progressive deterioration of the cartilage that is the hallmark of osteoarthritis.

"We have found the mechanism that begins to explain how and why aging leads to deterioration of articular cartilage," says Scripps Research Professor Martin Lotz, M.D., a world-renowned arthritis researcher. "Our findings demonstrate a direct link between the loss of this protein and osteoarthritis."

Stem cell transplantation for the study and treatment of osteoarthritis in humans is now being conducted at a few centers. The stem cells are autologous- meaning they are taken from a patient's own bone marrow.

They are then concentrated using a special technique. The area of injury at the site of knee osteoarthritis is then identified, "reinjured" using another special technique to induce an inflammatory response. Using ultrasound guidance, the stem cells are then introduced into the knee along with platelet-rich plasma, a component of whole blood, that stimulates receptors located on the surface of stem cells to cause multiplication and division of the stem cells.

While still investigational, the early results look promising. According to Dr. Nathan Wei, "We are measuring results using a number of devices including ultrasound measurement of cartilage thickness,

www.arthritistreatmentcenter.com

special x-ray views, health assessment questionnaires, and other similar tools."

He goes on to say, "One of the hurdles is that cartilage growth is slow. Often subjective measures of effectiveness, such as pain, improve much more quickly than objective measurements. We are still trying to develop specific profiles of patients that will determine which people are the best candidates. For instance, patients above the ages of 70-75 may not be the best candidates because of "sluggish" stem cell response. Also, obese people are definitely not candidates, so body mass index is an important selection criterion."

www.arthritistreatmentcenter.com

Chapter 6

If an earthworm can grow a new body, why can't a human grow new cartilage for their knee or hip?

If a tadpole's tail is cut off, it will grow a new one. If a salamander's leg is cut off, it will grow a new one. If an earthworm is cut in half, it will eventually grow a new half. If a snail's head is cut off, it will grow a new one. (Osborn HF, Wilson EB. Regeneration. Columbia University Biological Series. Macmillan Company. 1901)

Regeneration in lower forms of animals has been known about for at least a century in the scientific community. The primary reason lower forms of animals are able to regenerate lost limbs while higher forms such as humans can't, has been the subject of much conjecture. The most reasonable explanations include:

1. Stem cells in lower forms of animals are plentiful and available in sufficient concentrations to hasten regeneration.

2. Stem cells are in closer proximity- meaning that these animals have very simple organs that aren't nearly as compartmentalized as those of higher animal forms. What this means is that once a cell has differentiated into a heart cell or lung cell, it is committed. It cannot reverse the process. And, since stem cells are not that plentiful in the normal bloodstream

of higher animal forms such as humans, the ability to regenerate lost tissues is limited.

3. Finally, the amount of differentiation of cells into more complex and different types of organs is not quite so pronounced in earthworms and salamanders as compared with higher forms of animals. Brains, heart, and lung tissue are highly developed, very complex organs. And... these organs are located far away from a large supply of stem cells, since stem cells are rarely found in the peripheral blood. An earthworm or salamander doesn't have to worry about this problem!

Mammals do have the ability to "regenerate" to the extent that most wounds will heal over time.

However, the ability to heal degenerative processes or to manufacture new organs has been an elusive target.

At least until recently... it turns out that stem cells, the progenitor cells of all cells in the body, are what allow massive healing to take place. (By progenitor, I mean that stem cells are capable of differentiating into any type of organ cell.)

In higher mammals such as humans, the number of stem cells required for massive regeneration is not available under normal circumstances.

Stem cells are sparse in the general blood circulation. They are present within bone marrow where they are called "mesenchymal stem cells."

However, in the adult, even in the bone marrow, stem cells need to be concentrated in order to be effective for tissue regenerative processes.

The lack of sufficient stem cells in peripheral tissues as well as the absence of triggering mechanisms which can send the stem cells into the "warp speed" required to help with regeneration also aren't present under normal circumstances.

It is this relative lack and access to stem cells that has presented researchers with the problem of how to produce the same kind of healing in human beings as is seen in lower forms of animals.

Recent development in stem cell biology has shown much promise.

For instance, autologous stem cells (cells obtained directly from the patient) have been used to help heal an ailing heart (National Geographic, July 2008). And in a more recent article (Parade Magazine, September 28, 2008), investigators at the Hospital for Special Surgery in New York City have mentioned the possible application of stem cells and platelet-rich plasma in the treatment of arthritis.

It appears that a number of requirements must be met in order for the magic of stem cells to take hold for conditions such as osteoarthritis.

First, a large number of stem cells are required. This involves taking stem cells from the bone marrow of the patient and concentrating them.

Second, the stem cells must be viable, meaning the concentration process cannot damage the stem cells.

Third, a "trigger" such as platelet-rich plasma must be provided in order for certain substances such as growth hormone to stimulate the stem cells to replicate and differentiate.

Fourth, the arthritis area must be prepared properly. That means "injury" must be induced. Injury should be sufficient to induce stem cells to proliferate and differentiate but not enough to render stem cell therapy useless. In other words, special techniques need to be applied.

www.arthritistreatmentcenter.com

Fifth, the stem cells and platelet-rich plasma must be introduced in such a fashion that a framework or scaffold is prepared so that stem cells have a place to "latch onto" so they can accomplish what needs to be done.

A small number of centers in the U.S. are working on such a procedure. Early results look promising.

According to Dr. Nathan Wei, "Stem cell research is probably the future of treatment for osteoarthritis. We have to work on newer and better techniques... and also provide data that can be used to assess the efficacy of this type of therapy. To date we have treatments that help with symptoms... but we need therapies that can actually regrow cartilage and other damaged connective tissue.

Currently, we are in the middle of some very interesting work that looks very encouraging. The results are in the preliminary stages, so while the early evidence is extremely promising, longer term data is needed.

We are harvesting and concentrating mesenchymal stem cells. We are also providing a scaffold for stem cells to proliferate and grow.

Unfortunately, cartilage tissue grows relatively slowly... but we have to be patient. If the objective evidence- thickening... or growth of cartilage- matches the symptomatic improvement we've seen, this will be a major breakthrough!"

www.arthritistreatmentcenter.com

Chapter 7

What else can we learn from animals?

A study published recently (Grigolo B, et al. Osteoarthritis treated with mesenchymal stem cells on hyaluronan-based scaffold in rabbit. Tissue Engineering. 15; 2009: 1-4) described a rabbit model of osteoarthritis. Rabbit joints were subjected to cutting of the anterior cruciate ligament which induced osteoarthritis. After the eight-week period allowed for development of the disease, half the rabbits received mesenchymal stem cells seeded onto a hyaluronan scaffold. Untreated rabbits were used as controls. While all the animals developed osteoarthritis, statistically significant differences in the quality of the regenerated tissue were found when the animals with the scaffolds were compared to the animals who didn't receive the stem cells.

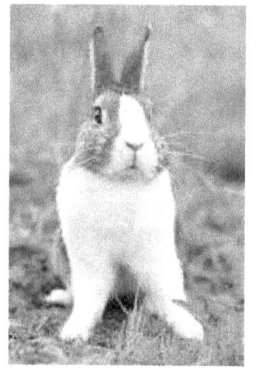

Veterinarians have aggressively tested new treatments for the most common injuries in race horses because these animals are so valuable and because these injuries can be so incapacitating. "Soft tissue injuries can end a race horse's career," states Dr. Sean Owens, a veterinarian and director of the Regenerative Medicine Laboratory at the University of California, Davis.

Veterinary medicine, unlike human medicine, is more permissive when it comes to experimental therapies, allowing these treatments to move more quickly into clinical use. Nonetheless, the focus of the

Davis center is on clinical trials modeled after those done in humans. The major difference is that at Davis, the patients are horses.

A company named VetCell, located in the United Kingdom, has prepared a stem cell product that has been used in 1,700 horses. In a study of 170 jumping horses, researchers showed that nearly 80 percent of them could return to competition compared with 30 percent given conventional treatment. After three years, the re-injury rate was much lower in the stem cell treated group as well. While the exact mechanism by which the stem cells work on soft tissue injuries is unknown, preliminary studies indicate the stem cells help tissue regenerate without forming scar tissue.

VetStem, a California-based company uses stem cells isolated from fat rather than bone marrow. A placebo-controlled study has shown that

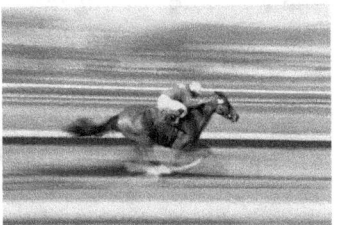 this treatment is helpful for dogs.

Another company, Cytori, also isolates stem cells from fat and may be planning to move into human clinical trials.

Chapter 8

Osteoarthritis: Are stem cells really the answer?

Osteoarthritis (OA) is the most common form of arthritis. In fact, it has been estimated that more than 100, 000 Americans cannot transfer from their beds to the bathroom as a result of osteoarthritis of the hip or knee.

The burden of OA is made worse by the inadequacies of current therapies.

Non-drug and various drug treatments are used for early OA, but protection of articular cartilage has so far not been available. Surgical intervention- meaning joint replacement- is often indicated when the symptoms cannot be controlled and the disease progresses.

A potentially valuable tool has been multipotent adult mesenchymal stem cells (MSCs), obtained from the bone marrow of normal adults. Many strategies have been studied and developed to possibly harness the ability of MSCs to differentiate into cartilage cells.

Osteoarthritis is a complicated disease. Cartilage cells, called chondrocytes, produce and secrete enzymes, such as matrix metalloproteinases and aggrecanases, which corrode and erode cartilage.

Interleukin 1 (IL-1) is an inflammatory chemical messenger which makes these enzymes cause more damage. Stimulation of these factors leads to damage to cartilage through both reduced synthesis as well as accelerated breakdown. Other inflammatory messengers such as tumor necrosis factor are also involved in cartilage breakdown and, along with mechanical factors, lead to worsening of the disease.

Despite much research into development of inhibitors of these molecules for use in treating OA, success with prevention of cartilage breakdown or with cartilage restoration has not been achieved.

That is why MSCs have been attractive. MSCs are cells that can be stimulated to differentiate along specific pathways, including cartilage production. In contrast to existing cartilage tissue which needs to be surgically harvested from non-weightbearing cartilage, MSCs can be harvested from bone marrow.

Some evidence exists that tissue damage in osteoarthritis is due to depletion of MSC populations.

So why haven't MSCs been used for OA treatment already?

First, questions exist as to whether MSCs obtained from patients with OA differ functionally from those of healthy people.

Also, age-dependent decline in the differentiation capability of MSCs has been reported by some investigators.

However, it should be pointed out that when MSCs are harvested and concentrated properly, enough MSCs with adequate differentiation potential can be isolated from patients with OA, irrespective of their age or the cause of their disease. These results indicate that MSCs for regeneration of cartilage in patients with OA is practical as well as feasible.

How to deliver stem cells is the biggest question. Direct into-the-joint injection of MSCs is, technically, the simplest approach to OA

www.arthritistreatmentcenter.com

therapy. Unfortunately, there is no guarantee and even less data to support the effectiveness of this approach.

Compared with direct into-the-joint injection, MSC application to cartilage surfaces using a scaffold offers more control. The scaffold may consist of either natural or synthetic material. (The scaffold technique is the one advocated and used at our center.)

Another possible approach: MSCs can be introduced with various viral vectors. This permits delivery of genes that encode proteins that could potentially reverse some of the damage in OA.

Chapter 9

Stem cell treatment for osteoarthritis of the knees and hips... can it work?

OA is a disease of weight-bearing joints such as the neck, low back, hips, and knees.

Glucosamine and chondroitin preparations have demonstrated a modest effect in the maintenance of cartilage... but studies have demonstrated conflicting evidence in regards to the quantity of improvement.

Recently, though, there has been increased interest in the use of stem cells as a possible treatment modality for this disease.

The use of fetal stem cells is highly controversial... however, there is another good source that escapes the controversy- adult stem cells.

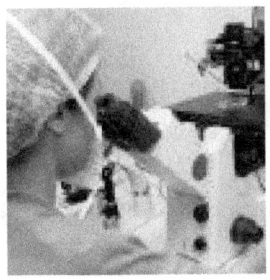

So what are stem cells? They are progenitor cells, meaning they are the earliest form of cell. Stem cells (SC) are manufactured in the bone marrow and are pluripotential. This means they can differentiate into any kind of tissue cell. Stem cells are responsible for growth and healing in the body.

The adult type is embryo-free and can create a specific body part, such as tissue, cartilage and bone.

www.arthritistreatmentcenter.com

So how are adult stem cells obtained? Adult stem cells are harvested from the posterior iliac crest of the pelvis (the back of the pelvis.) Using local anesthetic with ultrasound guidance, a small biopsy needle is introduced. A syringe is connected to the needle and is used to remove stem cells from the bone marrow. The stem cells are then prepared and concentrated using a technique involving a specially designed centrifuge.

At the same time blood is drawn from the patient in order to isolate platelet-rich plasma. This platelet-rich plasma contains specific growth factors that promote the regeneration of collagen, a major constituent of cartilage.

A small needle will be introduced into the knee using local anesthetic and "tease" the cartilage and the tendons that are the source of the arthritis … as well as the source of much of the pain- all under ultrasound guidance. An injection of stem cells and platelet-rich plasma will follow.   The end result is cartilage regeneration.

According to most experts, potential side effects are minimal. Most patients are surprised at how quickly they are active again. The advantage of stem cell therapy is that it's like getting a new set of tires. Unlike getting a knee replacement, you can go back to aerobics and running.

The advantage to stem cell therapy is that the patient is his/her own donor and provides his/her own therapy. It's a lot like giving a blood transfusion to yourself.

Because the cells aren't foreign to the body, engineered or manipulated in any way, there's no chance for contamination or rejection when the isolated cells re-enter the body.

www.arthritistreatmentcenter.com

This procedure is best for patients in the 30-70 year age range. When patients are older, their chondrocytes- cartilage cells- don't respond as well to stimulation by the stem cells and platelet-rich plasma.

Chapter 10

The ultimate betrayal of the knee arthritis lambs

About 20% of the 900,000 arthroscopic knee surgeries performed annually in North America are done as treatment for osteoarthritis (Time, 2008). A knee arthroscopy is a procedure where a small telescope is inserted into the joint and debris is removed. The vast majority are done by orthopedic surgeons.

It turns out that knee arthroscopy may be no more effective over two years than non-surgical treatment using physical therapy and medications, according to a recent study published in the New England Journal of Medicine (Kirkley A, et al. A Randomized Trial of Arthroscopic Surgery for Osteoarthritis of the Knee. NEJM. 2008; 359:1097-1107).

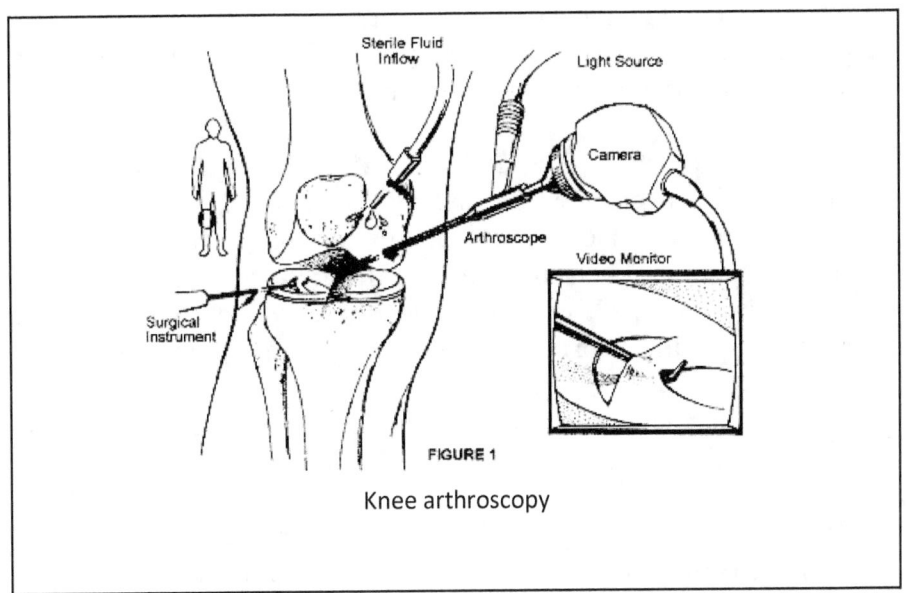

FIGURE 1

Knee arthroscopy

The researchers examined 178 patients who had an average age of 60. All patients received standard non-surgical treatment, including physical therapy, anti-inflammatory drugs or analgesics such as acetaminophen and ibuprofen, glucosamine supplements, and injections to lubricate the joint.

Eighty-six of the patients also underwent arthroscopic surgery. Patients were evaluated over two years using a scoring system that measured pain, stiffness and physical function. After three months, the surgery group initially showed more improvement, but two years after the procedure, there was no significant difference between the groups.

The results paralleled the findings of a 2002 Department of Veteran Affairs study conducted at the Houston VA (Moseley JB, et al. A Controlled Trial of Arthroscopic Surgery for Osteoarthritis of the Knee. NEJM. 2002; 347: 81-88).

www.arthritistreatmentcenter.com

In response to the most recent study, E. Anthony Rankin, MD, president of the American Academy of Orthopedic Surgeons, said, "As a tool for treating arthritis alone, it probably isn't a good tool."

In an accompanying editorial, Robert Marx, an orthopedic surgeon at the Cornell University Medical College of Cornell University, wrote that the study provides "strong support" for the conclusion that "arthroscopic surgery is not effective therapy for advanced osteoarthritis of the knee." Marx added that the procedure could offer benefits for patients experiencing additional knee problems.

Both orthopedic surgeons added that "knee replacement surgery is an option for those with serious arthritis."

Approximately 555,000 total knee replacement procedures, also called total knee arthroplasty (TKA), are performed each year (Saletan W. Washington Post September 14, 2008).

Primary total knee replacement is most commonly performed for osteoarthritis (OA).

So... orthopedic surgeons win no matter what. Surgeons perform surgery.

If they can't 'scope' a patient, they can replace the knee.

So what are the options for a patient if they don't want a knee replacement?

The big question is this: can cartilage – the gristle that caps the ends of long bones, and which wears away during the process of arthritis, re-grow? Some physicians like K. Dean Reeves, a physical medicine and rehabilitation specialist, in Kansas City, Kansas are studying the effects of prolotherapy in inducing cartilage growth.

www.arthritistreatmentcenter.com

Prolotherapy is a procedure where cartilage is purposefully injured to stimulate the formation of chondroblasts, early cartilage cells that have the ability to regenerate.

Dr. Reeves has just completed a double-blind study on knee arthritis using prolotherapy techniques.

In the knee arthritis study, after one year, there was a 44 percent improvement in pain, 63 percent improvement in swelling, and a 14-degree improvement in flexibility. There was an 85 percent reduction in knee buckling episodes. Improvement in joint space was also noted.

Other physicians are studying the effects of growth hormone.

Finally, the most promising approach appears to be the use of a combination of cartilage irritation and stem cells.

Currently, studies are being conducted studying the effects of a prolotherapy-like procedure in combination with autologous stem cells and growth factors for osteoarthritis of the knee. Autologous stem cells are stem cells obtained directly from the bone marrow of the patient. These stem cells are then concentrated using a special technique. Once they are reintroduced into the knee capsule along with other growth factors using ultrasound guidance, they have the capacity to differentiate into cartilage cells. Growth factors are used to send the healing phase into 'warp speed'.

The early results are very encouraging and parallel the findings of others. In the final analysis, if we can demonstrate significant improvements in clinical measures along with cartilage regeneration, we can reduce the tremendous number of knee surgeries performed every year.

If a patient has severe arthritis, "bone on bone," with no cartilage left, then this procedure is not going to be helpful. That patient will most

www.arthritistreatmentcenter.com

likely need a knee replacement. It's important to see the patient before this stage.

Chapter 11

How stem cells are delivered

A requirement for mesenchymal stem cell (MSC) therapy for osteoarthritis is the delivery of the cells to the defected site. Direct into-the-joint injection might be possible in early stages of the disease when the defect is restricted to the cartilage layer, whereas a scaffold or matrix of some kind would be required to support the MSCs in cases where the bone underneath the cartilage is exposed over large areas.

Direct into-the-joint injection of MSCs is the easiest approach to OA therapy. After injection, MSCs would spread throughout the joint space, and would interact with any receptive cells and surfaces. The synovium lines the joint space and is packed with cells. It would probably interact with MSCs.

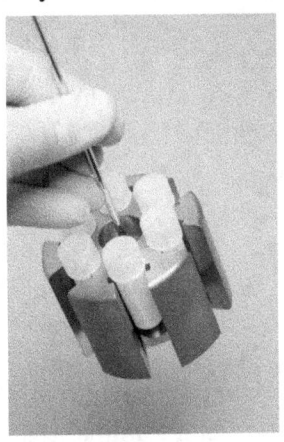

Preparing stem cells for injection

Direct joint injection of MSCs has been studied in animal models. In one study, autologous MSCs in a solution of hyaluronic acid were injected into the knee joints of goats, in which OA had been induced surgically (Murphy JM *et al.* Stem cell therapy in a caprine model of osteoarthritis. *Arthritis Rheum.*2003; 48: 3464-3474).

Joints exposed to MSCs showed evidence of regeneration. Articular cartilage degeneration, spur remodeling, and bone abnormalities were also reduced in the treated joints.

In another study, a cartilage defect in the knee joints of mini-pigs was also treated by direct injection of MSCs suspended in hyaluronic acid into the joint (Lee KB *et al.* Injectable mesenchymal stem cell therapy for large cartilage defects--a porcine model. *Stem Cells.* 2007; 25: 2964-2971).

The treated animals showed improved cartilage healing compared with the control group.

The exact mechanisms that guide MSCs to the areas of damage are not known, but it is clear that these cells secrete a broad spectrum of bioactive molecules that have immunoregulatory properties (Chen X *et al.* Mesenchymal stem cells in immunoregulation. *Immunol Cell Biol.* 2006; 84: 413-421) and/or regenerative activities (Kan I *et al.* Autotransplantation of bone marrow-derived stem cells as a therapy for neurodegenerative diseases. *Handb Exp Pharmacol.* 2007; 180: 219-242).

Bioactive factors produced by MSCs have been shown to prevent tissue scarring, suppress cellular death, stimulate blood vessel growth, and increase the production of stem cells.

Compared with direct joint injection, using a scaffold offers more control. Introducing MSCs via a scaffold, offers the advantage of an easy-to-manipulate, self-renewing source of stem cells.

Mesenchymal stem cells could be grown into a glue-like scaffold or a customized mold (like a puzzle piece) before being implanted into the damaged area of cartilage.

The ideal scaffold should be biocompatible and biodegradable, porous to permit cell penetration and tissue impregnation, permeable to allow nutrient delivery and gas exchange, and adaptable to the mechanical environment (Noth U, Steinert AF, Tuan RS. Technology Insight: Adult Mesenchymal Stem Cells for Osteoarthritis Therapy. Nat Clin Pract Rheumatol. 2008;4 (7):371-380).

Synthetic scaffolds have been designed. Many synthetic scaffolds used are made using α-hydroxy polyesters. A recent example is a nanofibrous scaffold of biodegradable polymers which has demonstrated enhanced support of MSC growth and differentiation (Li WJ *et al*. Application of nanofibrous scaffolds in skeletal tissue engineering. *J Biomed Nanotechnol*. 2005; 1: 1-17).

Natural materials, composed of collagen, fibrin, and hyaluronon offer the advantage of being biodegradable, offer a natural environment that leads to rapid attachment of cells, and are less likely to induce an inflammatory response. (Kuo CK *et al*. Cartilage tissue engineering: its potential and uses. *Curr Opin Rheumatol* . 2006; 18: 64-73). So, the bottom line is they provide a more natural microenvironment for MSCs than synthetic scaffolds do.

The first results for use of transplanted MSCs seeded within collagen type I hydrogels to repair isolated, full-thickness, cartilage defects in humans have been reported (Wakitani S *et al*. Autologous bone marrow stromal cell transplantation for repair of full-thickness articular cartilage defects in human patellae: two case reports. *Cell Transplant*. 2004; 13: 595-600).

Two patients with a patellar defect were treated with collagen gels containing MSCs, which were covered with a periosteal flap. Fibrocartilaginous filling of the defects was found after 1 year, and both patients showed significantly improved clinical outcomes in their follow-ups after 1, 4, and 5 years.

The same group (Kuroda R *et al*. Treatment of a full-thickness articular cartilage defect in the femoral condyle of an athlete with autologous bone-marrow stromal cells. *Osteoarthritis Cartilage.* 2007; 15: 226-231) also used this protocol to treat another patient with a full-thickness cartilage defect in the weight-bearing area of the medial femoral condyle. The patient's clinical symptoms had improved significantly 1 year after surgery. Examination under the microscope showed the defect was filled with a hyaline-like type of cartilage tissue.

These pilot studies have been performed on isolated or focal articular cartilage defects in an otherwise healthy joint. The abnormalities of cartilage metabolism that occur in OA create a very different environment, which will influence MSC engraftment and tissue differentiation. The potential outcome of matrix-based cell transplantation in an OA joint is still unclear (Nesic D *et al.* Cartilage tissue engineering for degenerative joint disease. *Adv Drug Deliv Rev.* 2006; 58: 300-322).

Another potential avenue is to use non-pathogenic viruses such as adeno-associated virus or lentivirus to transport genes to stem cells to promote growth and differentiation. Using this approach, stem cells can be directed to differentiate into cartilage cells and allow a more stable environment. Stem cells can therefore be programmed to express anti-inflammatory and pro-survival factors to combat the natural tendency for stem cells to die off from oxidative stress, and more importantly, program them not to proliferate into tumors.

Generally, cartilage lesions in OA are usually large, unconfined, and affect more than one location.

They are frequently accompanied by a varus or valgus deformity. The direct pressure on the transplanted cells creates a high probability that implanted matrices will be rapidly worn down as a result of joint movement. This indicates the need for limited weight-bearing and the use of unloading devices to minimize stress on the newly treated joint.

www.arthritistreatmentcenter.com

And this also supports the role of gene transfer as a viable and attractive model for the future. Cell suspensions of virally transformed stem cells can be sent to repair diseased cartilage and replace lost chondrocytes through continual expression of chondrogenic, anti-inflammatory, and pro-survival genes.

Chapter 12

Doctor... I don't want a joint replacement for my arthritis. What are my options?

While the treatment of end-stage OA of weight-bearing joints such as the hips and knees has been enhanced by surgical joint replacement techniques, joint surgery also has its many downsides including complications related to the procedure, complications arising from anesthesia, and the hefty price tag associated with the procedure which is a drag on the healthcare system.

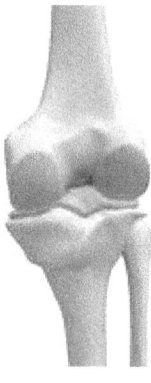

Knee joint

A recent study done by researchers at Florida International University analyzed increases in surgeries and costs between 1997 and 2004. The April 2008 issue of Arthritis Care & Research presents eyebrow-raising numbers that conclude with the author's contention that "the burden resulting from hip/knee joint replacement is not only substantial but also increasing at a steep rate."

Among the findings include:

- In 2004, approximately 431,485 primary knee replacements were performed, a 53 percent increase from the year 2000. 225,900 primary hip replacements were performed in the US, marking a 37 percent increase for the same period.

www.arthritistreatmentcenter.com

50

- In 1997, about 60 percent of primary hip replacements and 69 percent of primary knee replacements were performed on individuals between the ages of 65 and 84 years. Although elderly patients remained the main recipients, the number of joint replacement surgeries among the middle-aged patients between 45 and 64 years, increased excessively, 71 percent for hip replacements and 83 percent for knee replacements in 2004.
- Between 1997 and 2004, the hospital charges for joint replacements, both primary and revision surgeries, increased faster than the rate of inflation. While Medicare continued to provide the principal source of payment, compared with other sources of payment, the relative burden decreased. The burden on private insurance more than tripled in that 7-year span from $1.1 billion to $3 billion for hip replacements and from $1.46 billion to $4.64 billion for knee replacements.

According to the research, led by Dr. Sunny Kim, "If current trends persist, nearly 600,000 hip replacements and 1.4 million knee replacements will be performed in the year 2015."

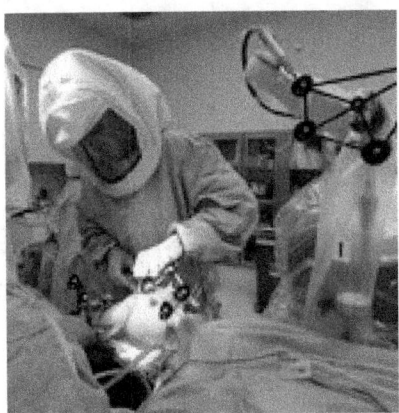

Knee replacement surgery

www.arthritistreatmentcenter.com

Dr. Kim and colleagues stressed the need for "public health education …to reduce the proportion of people who are overweight as well as to manage arthritis at earlier stages… the health care community should be prepared for this upcoming demand of surgical loads and its economic burden on government and private insurance systems."

These sobering statistics point towards the need for therapies designed to prolong the life of cartilage and possibly to regenerate new cartilage. While the thrust of research until recently has been to evaluate drugs that might have disease-modifying potential, clinical trial results have been disappointing.

In addition, stop-gap measures such as glucocorticoid ("cortisone") and viscosupplement (lubricant) injections may not provide long-term relief. In addition, glucocorticoids lead to more cartilage deterioration.

However, a new approach, ironically, borrowed from the veterinary sector, shows great promise in the possibility of cartilage regeneration.

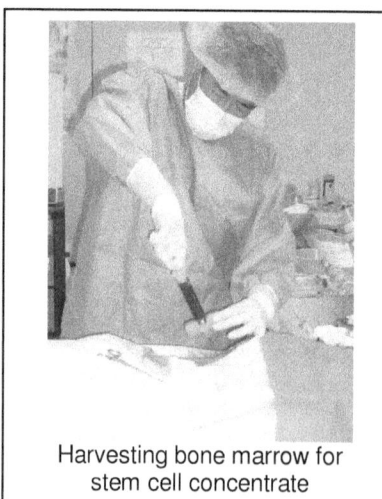

Harvesting bone marrow for stem cell concentrate

Stem cells are pluripotential cells, meaning they are capable of differentiating into any type of cell in the body, given the right circumstances. Orthopedic surgeons have been interested in designing tissue scaffold techniques to help preserve cartilage. However, the procedures are cumbersome and require recuperation periods of between 6 and 12 months.

It is now possible to harvest a person's own stem cells by using a small gauge biopsy needle inserted into the iliac crest (back of the pelvis). Stem cells are then concentrated.

At the same time, platelet-rich plasma is obtained from the patient's whole blood. Platelets are cells in the blood that contain multiple growth and healing factors.

A medium gauge needle is then inserted into the hip or knee and used to "irritate" the cartilage and adjacent tendons to stimulate an inflammatory response. Inflammation is the body's response to injury and is the first stage of healing. The stem cells and platelet-rich plasma are then injected into the joint and the patient is placed at limited weight-bearing for one week.

Follow-up imaging studies including magnetic resonance imaging and diagnostic ultrasound have confirmed the re-growth of cartilage in small uncontrolled studies. These observations are consistent with the larger scale controlled studies seen in the veterinary literature.

Patient selection is important in that patients over the age of 75 tend to have "senescent chondrocytes." This means their cartilage cells are older and less responsive to stem cell stimulation. That is not meant to entirely exclude patients in their 70's. A patient who is physically active, at ideal weight, and is interested in remaining so, might be a much better candidate than a 50-year old couch potato.

The added attraction is that this procedure can be done in an outpatient facility at a fraction of the cost of a joint replacement!

www.arthritistreatmentcenter.com

Chapter 13

Knee replacement surgery may be a thing of the past for many Baby Boomers

Today, Baby Boomers (defined as those people born between the years 1946 to 1964) are living longer, staying more active, and are very interested in continuing to maintain a vigorous lifestyle.

Multiple research studies have demonstrated the benefit of regular exercise in forestalling the complications related to such degenerative conditions as diabetes and Alzheimer's disease.

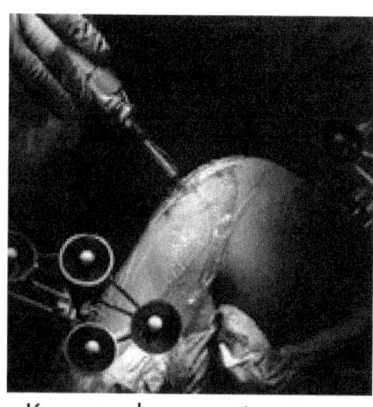

Knee replacement surgery

Exercise is also important in maintaining the health of joints by strengthening muscles, improving blood flow, and promoting joint flexibility.

Nonetheless, many people find, even as early as their 40's that they have significant problems with arthritis. They then go to see orthopedic surgeons who- as surgeons are trained to do- want to operate.

According to statistics provided by the American Academy of Orthopedic Surgeons, hip replacements in the United States are expected to double from 285,000 in 2005 to 572,000 in 2030, with

www.arthritistreatmentcenter.com

knee replacements also shooting through the roof from 523,000 to 3.4 million over the same period of time.

Most joint replacement operations are performed for osteoarthritis, the most common form of arthritis. While newer techniques for joint replacement are making this operation more attractive, what can a Baby Boomer who has OA but who doesn't want joint replacement surgery to do?

Standard conservative therapies consist of weight control, regular exercise, and avoidance of activities that aggravate symptoms.

For pain control, analgesics such as acetaminophen (Tylenol) and various non-steroidal anti-inflammatory drugs (NSAIDS) are sometimes helpful. Unfortunately, they also have the potential for harmful side effects. Topical non-steroidal drugs may be preferable.

For patients with more severe symptoms, injections of glucocorticoids ("cortisone") and viscosupplements, which are special lubricants, can alleviate pain.

Devices such as lateral wedge insoles worn in shoes to realign the knee or unloader-type braces can also be useful for some.

In patients with significant discomfort who still have cartilage left, there is another option. Born of the regenerative medicine movement, resurgent interest in the use of autologous stem cells (stem cells obtained from the patient), has prompted the development of new treatment approaches.

One such approach is the use of autologous stem cells along with platelet-rich plasma (platelets are blood cells rich in healing and growth factors) to help grow new cartilage.

www.arthritistreatmentcenter.com

One other surgical option that is relatively popular is joint resurfacing particularly for younger patients with osteoarthritis of the hip. The data is still pending.

Chapter 14

Osteoarthritis of the knee... A young person's disease

Osteoarthritis (OA) is the type of arthritis that conjures up the picture of an elderly person who has aches and pains.

New data though shows that osteoarthritis begins earlier, probably in the second decade, in many patients.

Dr. Ewa Roos, professor in the Institute of Sports Science and Clinical Biomechanics of the University of Southern Denmark, presented an intriguing paper outlining her research. In it she described two populations of patients who suffer from osteoarthritis of the knee. The first group was comprised mainly of older women. The other group, though, consisted of men in their 30's and 40's (Roos EM, et al. Arthritis Rheum 2005; 52: 3507-3514).

A major hurdle to early diagnosis is that many younger patients with symptoms will have negative imaging studies... in other words, x-rays and magnetic resonance imaging (MRI) tests will be normal.

To complicate matters, patients who have x-ray evidence of osteoarthritis don't necessarily have symptoms.

Risk factors that are common to people with osteoarthritis are genetic predisposition and excessive weight.

In addition, patients who have suffered knee injuries to the anterior cruciate ligament (ACL) and menisci- the cartilage cushions in the knee- are also at increased risk for developing OA (Englund M, et al. Arthritis Rheum 2007; 56:4048-4054).

In related studies, it has been shown that regular exercise is both protective and preventative as far as osteoarthritis of the knee is concerned.

In other words, exercise appears to strengthen joint cartilage in patients with OA of the knee. Measurements of glycosaminoglycans, an indicator of strength and elasticity in the joint, showed significant improvements in the knees of patients with OA who regularly exercised compared to control subjects who did not.

Many patients with OA of the knees are resistant to the idea of exercise since they feel it may cause the joints to wear down even faster. The results of the above studies clearly indicate that exercise should be encouraged.

For symptomatic relief, strengthening and stretching exercises accompanied by the judicious use of ice and anti-inflammatory medications may be quite helpful.

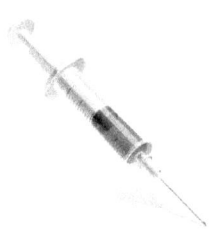

www.arthritistreatmentcenter.com

In the past, corticosteroid ("cortisone") injections were routinely prescribed for patients with moderate to severe pain from OA. However, evidence indicating that corticosteroids ultimately cause cartilage to wear away faster than it should, has concerned physicians to the point where these injections are used less.

Viscosupplements, lubricants that help the knee to glide better, and which may help slow down the process of wear and tear are beneficial for some patients.

More recently, the use of autologous stem cell therapy (stem cells harvested from the patient himself) has shown great promise, not only for symptomatic relief but for actual reversal of cartilage wear and tear with possible re-growth of cartilage.

Resurfacing procedures may be advisable for younger patients; however, the data is contradictory regarding the results of this surgical approach. Total joint replacement is reserved for those patients in whom conservative measures have failed.

Chapter 15

Stem cell therapy for arthritis: Is it possible to wind the aging clocks of the cartilage cells in your joints backwards?

Research on stem cells is leading scientists to investigate the possibility of cell-based therapies to treat disease, an area which is often referred to as regenerative medicine.

Stem cells have two important characteristics that distinguish them from other types of cells. First, they are unspecialized cells that renew themselves for long periods of time through cell division. The second is that under certain physiologic or experimental conditions, they can be induced to become cells with special functions.

There are two different sources of stem cells. Embryonic cells are derived from fetal tissue and are a source of great controversy. Adult stem cells (ASC), on the other hand, are found in normal people.

ASC can renew themselves, and can differentiate to yield the major specialized cell types of the tissue or organ. Their primary role in a living organism is to maintain and repair the tissue in which they are found.

Research on adult stem cells has recently generated a great deal of excitement. Scientists have found adult stem cells in many more tissues than they once thought possible. This finding has led scientists to ask whether adult stem cells could be used for transplants. In fact, adult blood-forming stem cells from bone marrow have been used in transplants for 30 years. Certain kinds of adult stem cells seem to have the ability to differentiate into a number of different cell types, given the proper conditions.

Bone marrow derived stem cells give rise to a variety of cell types: bone cells (osteocytes), cartilage cells (chondrocytes), fat cells (adipocytes), and other kinds of connective tissue cells such as those in tendons.

According to information from the National Institutes of Health, "One of the fundamental properties of a stem cell is that it does not have any tissue-specific structures that allow it to perform specialized functions. Unlike muscle cells, blood cells, or nerve cells, which do not normally replicate themselves, stem cells may replicate many times.

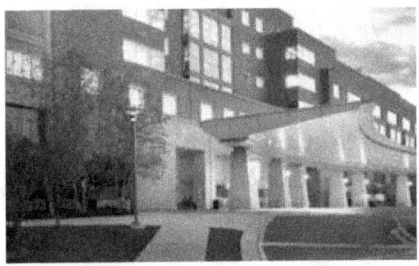

Clinical Center, National Institutes of Health,
Bethesda, Maryland

When cells replicate themselves many times over it is called proliferation. A starting population of stem cells that proliferates for many months in the laboratory can yield millions of cells."

The process by which unspecialized stem cells become specialized cells is called differentiation. Adult stem cells typically generate the cell types of the tissue in which they reside. A blood-forming adult

www.arthritistreatmentcenter.com

stem cell in the bone marrow, for example, normally gives rise to the various types of blood cells such as red blood cells, white blood cells and platelets. Until recently, it had been thought that a blood-forming cell in the bone marrow could not give rise to the cells of a very different tissue.

However, a number of experiments over the last several years have raised the possibility that stem cells from one tissue may be able to give rise to cell types of a completely different tissue. This phenomenon is referred to as "plasticity."

Two recent research presentations shore up the promise of stem cells in arthritis. First, research presented in April 2008 at the United Kingdom National Stem Cell Network Annual Science Meeting in Edinburgh offered hope that stem cells may be harnessed to repair the damaged cartilage that is responsible for the main symptoms of osteoarthritis.

On a related note, scientists at Cardiff University in the United Kingdom have successfully identified stem cells within articular cartilage of adults, which have the ability to become chondrocytes, cells that make up cartilage. The team has even been able to identify the cells in people over 75 years of age.

Lead researcher Professor Charlie Archer from the Cardiff School of Biosciences said:

"This research could have real benefits for arthritis sufferers and especially younger active patients with cartilage lesions that can progress to whole scale osteoarthritis."

The focus is on adult autologous stem cells ("autologous" meaning derived from the patient himself). These cells are present within a patient's bone marrow. Once we obtain the stem cells, they need to be concentrated using special techniques in order to secure the number of stem cells per unit volume needed. We have been using this treatment, combined with growth factors obtained from other cells, for both osteoarthritis of the knee as well as the hip.

Preliminary results using both subjective as well as objective measures show much promise. If these results are validated, the springtime of your life when it comes to weight-bearing joints may actually be 55-75.

Chapter 16

I look ten years younger since my facelift… but my knees still feel their age… What can I do?

One of the first mentions of stem cell therapy for osteoarthritis was an article published in the December 2003 issue of Arthritis and Rheumatism (Murphy JM, et al. Arthritis Rheum. 2003; 48: 3464-3474.)

The research team took two groups of goats and created osteoarthritis in their knees by removing the medial meniscus and cutting out the anterior cruciate ligament. After six weeks, one group of goats received an injection of sodium hyaluronan (a lubricant commonly used to treat symptomatic osteoarthritis of the knee) while the other group received a single dose of 10 million stem cells, originally extracted from the goats' bone marrow, and then suspended in sodium hyaluronan before injection into the knee.

In the knees which had been treated by stem cell injections, researchers observed a regeneration of joint tissue and a decrease in cartilage degeneration.

The authors commented on their findings… "There may be a therapeutic benefit associated with local delivery of stem cells following traumatic injury to the knee. The longer term effect of this may be a reduction or delay in the progression to osteoarthritis."

The authors concluded that "This is a scaffold-free method for cell delivery and is therefore unencumbered by the complexities associated with placement of a solid cell construct." This latter statement is important because so many techniques to date have involved the complicated use of different scaffolds (frameworks) to hold stem cells in place.

Stem cells are progenitor cells—the cells that all others are derived from. They have three interesting characteristics that make them prime candidates for tissue regenerative techniques. They are capable of dividing and renewing their numbers for an unusually long period of time; they are undifferentiated, meaning they have not yet committed to being a "heart" cell or a "lung" cell; and they can become any type of specialized cell. Another term to refer to this property is that stem cells are "pluripotential."

While most research and ethical concerns have been centered on the use of embryonic stem cells, adult stem cells are more accessible with no ethical "baggage." The cells that were used in the above study were adult stem cells obtained from the bone marrow.

www.arthritistreatmentcenter.com

Chapter 17

Who's a good candidate for stem cell treatment for knee osteoarthritis?

In the early part of December 2009, the Vatican issued a pronouncement, again condemning the use of embryonic stem cells for medical research and medical treatment.

While this proclamation will hinder the development of some therapies in medicine, it should not be a major stumbling block in the management of osteoarthritis.

The reason?

Current approaches using stem cells for osteoarthritis are able to make use of autologous stem cells. These are stem cells obtained from the iliac crest (hip) of the patient using a special biopsy needle.

Stem cells are located within the bone marrow. The iliac crest is an ideal site for harvesting bone marrow. Since the procedure is done using local anesthetic, the risks of the procedure are minimal.

Autologous stem cells have the ability to differentiate into other tissue cells. Previously, it was felt this trait was not possible for adult stem cells; however, it has been confirmed that stem cells harvested from an adult are capable of differentiation.

www.arthritistreatmentcenter.com

Once the stem cells are harvested, they are concentrated using a special technique. In addition, platelet-rich plasma which is derived from a patient's whole blood is also obtained. Platelets are cells that contain numerous growth and healing properties. These growth factors have the ability to fire off tyrosine kinase receptors on the surface of stem cells and accelerate differentiation and multiplication.

The joint, usually the knee or hip, is then prepared by "irritating" the cartilage using a special biopsy needle. After this, stem cells and platelet-rich plasma are introduced into the joint.

Calcium chloride and thrombin as well as subcutaneous fat are also used to create a "scaffold" for the stem cells to locate themselves.

Diagnostic ultrasound is used throughout to ensure the proper location for harvesting the stem cells as well as the best location for introducing the stem cells into the target joint. The use of ultrasound is mandatory for proper anatomic placement!

So who might be a candidate for this procedure?

First, it's important to realize that a patient must have some cartilage remaining in the joint for stem cells to do their job.

Let's take the example of osteoarthritis of the knee. Osteoarthritis is currently graded in clinical trials using standing knee x-rays to quantify the amount of cartilage present within the knee.

The Kellgren-Lawrence classification is used. Grade 1 means the amount of cartilage is relatively normal. Grade 4 means that the patient is "bone on bone." Patients who are Kellgren- Lawrence Grade 4 are generally not considered candidates for stem cell treatment. Patients who are grades 1-3 are acceptable.

www.arthritistreatmentcenter.com

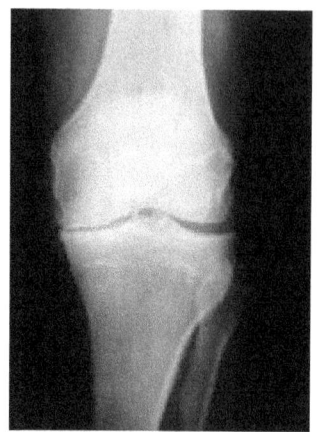
Knee x-ray Kellgren-Lawrence 4

Patients who are grade 3 must be at or near ideal weight.

Age also plays a role. It appears that as people get older, their stem cells respond less to stem cell stimulation. At our center, we generally use 75 as the cutoff. Even then the patient must be vigorous and active.

The ideal patient is between the ages of 30-70 and is at or near ideal weight. Healthy Baby Boomers who are athletic and active are felt to be the best candidates.

What measures are assessed?

We are currently evaluating both subjective as well as objective parameters. These include a visual analogue scale of pain, a Health Assessment Questionnaire (WOMAC), 50 foot walking time, knee x-rays done using special angulation to allow precise measurements of cartilage thickness, and ultrasound measurements of cartilage thickness.

The length of recovery is highly variable depending on factors such as age, general physical condition, Kellgren-Lawrence stage, and amount of "irritation" required to prepare the cartilage.

Chapter 18

Tissue engineering: An explanation of how stem cells can be used to regrow cartilage

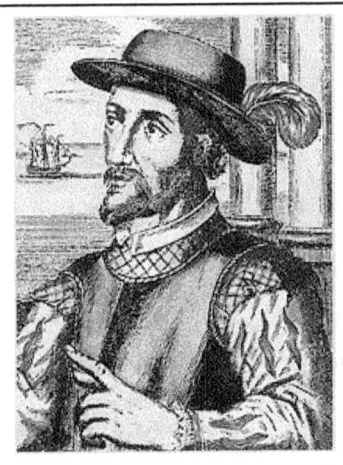

Ponce De Leon, Searcher of the Fountain of Youth

The perpetual search for the Fountain of Youth has both fascinated as well as eluded human beings for centuries.

What has been particularly interesting has been the observation that other species (i.e. earthworms, salamanders, etc.) can regenerate severed body parts… but human beings cannot.

The recent surge in interest in tissue engineering has been prompted by the scientific discoveries that perhaps the use of stem cell technology may allow a certain degree of tissue healing and regeneration to take place. Certainly, at least some of the impetus arises from the desire of Baby Boomers to remain active and healthy.

www.arthritistreatmentcenter.com

In the medical arena, there has been intense interest, particularly in the field of arthritis, regarding the potential use of stem cell technology to regrow cartilage.

It might be useful to quickly review what stem cells are and what types of stem cells might be used.

Stem cells are pluripotential progenitor cells. What this means is that these cells have not yet committed to become a specific type of tissue. Stem cells are the earliest type of cell. They have not yet "committed" to becoming a specific type of organ cell. However, given a specific stimulus, they can differentiate into any type of tissue. A heart cell… a lung cell… a brain cell… and so on.

There are three main types of stem cells that have been used in research to treat medical conditions.

The first are embryonic stem cells. These are obtained from a fetus. Of the three types of stem cells, embryonic stem cells are the cells that probably have the greatest potential to differentiate and multiply. However, there are concerns. Stem cells have been found to lead to cancer in at least one case of a boy who was given stem cells to treat a rare neurologic disorder. According to the Associated Press, "For all the promise, researchers have long warned that they must learn to control newly injected stem cells so they don't grow where they shouldn't, and small studies in people are only just beginning…" In addition, the ethical debate regarding the use of embryonic stem cells is also not over.

The second type of stem cell is called the mesenchymal donor cell. These are stem cells that are harvested from the bone marrow of normal volunteers. These have the potential to be quite useful. One advantage is that a large concentration of stem cells can be produced through this process. Questions still remain regarding the possibility of rejection reactions as well as the theoretical danger of transmission of viruses.

The most commonly used stem cells currently are autologous stem cells. These are stem cells that are obtained from the bone marrow of the patient. Stem cells by themselves may not be effective in differentiating into the tissue that is desired.

Stem cells are stimulated to multiply and divide as a result of having tyrosine kinase receptors on their surface which permit engagement with various growth factors. Growth factors present in blood, and in even higher concentration in platelet-rich plasma (PRP), bind to the tyrosine kinase receptors and send a signal to the nucleus of the cell that leads to replication.

In addition to these natural occurring growth factors, scientists are studying the ability of substances such as bone morphogenic protein (BMP) to stimulate bone and cartilage growth.

Also, in order for stem cells to replicate, they require a matrix which is capable of acting as a "home base." Different types of matrices form a framework in which stem cells can multiply and divide. Currently, scientists are studying various types of matrices to see which is the most effective.

From this discussion, it is quite clear that there are many questions that need to be addressed and answered. Regardless of the complexity of stem cell technology, it is clear that this area of regenerative medicine holds a great deal of promise for the future.

www.arthritistreatmentcenter.com

Chapter 19

More about stem cells and PRP for osteoarthritis

A number of methods have been used to repair cartilage damage. The first is osteochondral transplantation, which involves taking a plug of cartilage from a non-weight bearing area and placing it into a defect in a weight-bearing region. The second is microfracture. In this procedure, a surgeon will drill a number of small (2 mm diameter) holes into the cartilage until bleeding from the bone marrow occurs. The theory is that stem cells from the bone marrow will "leak out" and heal the cartilage damage. The final method is the use of autologous stem cell implantation with or without the assistance of a scaffold matrix to hold the cells.

The problem is that all these techniques have been used to treat focal cartilage lesions and not osteoarthritis. Also, recuperation from the first two procedures (chondral plug and microfracture) is exceedingly long.

Osteoarthritis lesions are generally large and unconfined and as a result may not hold onto chondrocytes (early cartilage cells) long enough for them to repair the damage.

Of the three methods described above, the one that seems to be garnering the most interest lately is autologous stem cells.

Results from a number of uncontrolled studies seem to show that stem cells can be harnessed to repair and possibly regenerate cartilage damage in OA.

Duke researchers have recently reported on their findings that stem cells obtained from the fat pad behind the kneecap can be reprogrammed to become cartilage cells. This research is preliminary but is worth noting.

Other theoretical problems and questions regarding the use of autologous stem cells include the following:

- Inability to get enough stem cells from the host
- The relative weakness of older stem cells to multiply and divide
- The possible metabolic abnormality in stem cells taken from a patient with osteoarthritis that might make them more susceptible to degrading earlier
- The inability to stimulate the stem cells to grow
- The best type of matrix to use to "house" the stem cells so they have a place to grow

Recent technological advances have enabled us to address these questions. Through the use of special techniques, harvesting a significant volume of bone marrow aspirate, then concentrating it into a small volume containing anywhere from 1-5 million stem cells has been easily accomplished.

While older stem cells may not have the growth potential of younger ones, they do appear to function well enough to regenerate connective tissue. Still, it is probably wise, in the patient selection process, to exclude patients above a certain age.

There is no convincing evidence that the stem cells obtained from patients with osteoarthritis contain a metabolic defect that would render them ineffective. Nonetheless, this area requires more research.

www.arthritistreatmentcenter.com

Stimulation of stem cell growth requires the use of growth factors that will bind to the tyrosine kinase receptors on the surface of stem cells. Once the receptors have been stimulated, a signal is sent to the nucleus of the stem cells leading to cell growth and proliferation.

The best "stimulant" appears to be platelet-rich plasma which is easily obtained from a patient's peripheral blood. Platelet-rich plasma (PRP) contains platelet-derived growth factor, transforming growth factor-B, fibrinogen, IL-1, epidermal growth factor, vascular endothelial growth factor, and adhesion molecules.

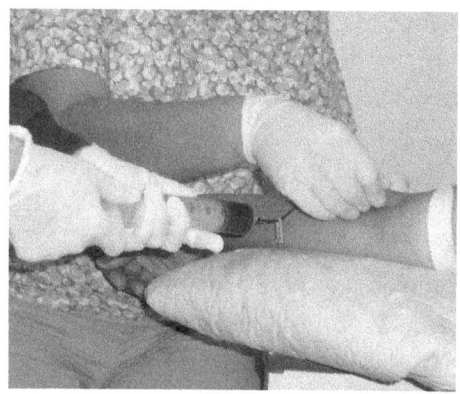

Drawing blood for preparation of PRP

This is a potent soup of protein messengers that readily attach to tyrosine kinase receptors located on stem cell surfaces. This causes a signal to be sent to the cell nucleus and causes the cell to multiply and divide.

A number of different matrices have been used and this area is still being explored. The major logistical problem is creating a matrix that is biocompatible, biodegradable, and easily instilled.

At our center we use a mixture of calcium chloride, thrombin, and fat, to create a gel that stem cells are bound to.

The joint is prepared using a specific approach designed to induce a local inflammatory response at the site to be healed. Autologous stem cells, PRP, and the matrix are then introduced carefully using ultrasound needle guidance.

To date, clinical response has been excellent.

www.arthritistreatmentcenter.com

Autologous stem cells provide an attractive option for both osteoarthritis patients and their physicians. Combining stem cells and PRP appears to be physiologically sound and more importantly, effective. This procedure holds much promise for Baby Boomers who wish to remain active.

www.arthritistreatmentcenter.com

Conclusion

As with all new technologies and treatments, more questions than answers exist.

For example:

What is the best and safest type of stem cell to use for osteoarthritis: embryonic, allogeneic, or autologous?

How do we ensure that unchecked growth (i.e. cancer) doesn't develop if embryonic stem cells are used?

How many stem cells need to be used for a given situation?

What type of quality control is required for stem cell harvesting as well as stem cell administration?

Is the best approach to treat regionally with multiple fenestrations (multiple passes with a needle to induce inflammation)? Is it necessary?

At what point should stem cells be used?

What's the best scaffold material to use?

Are other growth factors needed to help the stem cells perform better? If so, what kind? Currently, we are using platelet-rich plasma (PRP) but nothing else. Should we be using something else? If so, what and how much?

www.arthritistreatmentcenter.com

How does one deal with patients where a significant mechanical issue exists, e.g. varus (bowleg) or valgus (knock knee) deformities? It is quite evident to me at least that patients with significant mechanical problems need to have the treated joint rested for a significant length of time.

The answers to these questions and more, need to be answered before stem cell treatment for osteoarthritis becomes a mainstream therapy. However, everyday, at our center, we are working to address these issues and come up with practical solutions that will benefit our patients.

I hope you've enjoyed this book and I look forward to hearing from you.

For more information on stem cells and osteoarthritis contact us at:

Arthritis Treatment Center
71 Thomas Johnson Drive
Frederick, Maryland 21702
(301) 694 5800
(301) 694-0187 Fax
www.arthritistreatmentcenter.com

You may email me at: nwei@arthritistreatmentcenter.com

www.arthritistreatmentcenter.com

If you want to know more about stem cells, go to:
http://thebookonstemcellsforosteoarthritis.com/bookoffer/ (password: stem cell) our premium program on stem cell therapy.

Discover...

- The first sign of knee arthritis that should make you think of stem cells immediately... do you know what it is?
- How stem cells rebuild damaged joints organically, one cell at a time using a special "nutrient cocktail."
- Why sheep may be your best friend if you're thinking about stem cell therapy,
- Why most orthopedic surgeons just hate stem cells, and
- Who's the best candidate for stem cells... and who's the worst... find out now!

Get 20% off the regular price of the Stem Cell Program.

Copy the following link on to your internet browser to take advantage of these incredible savings!

http://thebookonstemcellsforosteoarthritis.com/bookoffer/
(password: stem cell)

www.arthritistreatmentcenter.com